The Rise of Plant-Based Diets:

"Why Veganism is Taking Over"

James E. Houck

Table of contents

- Health Benefits of Plant-Based Diets
- Environmental Implications
- Animal Welfare and Ethical Considerations
- Celebrity Endorsements and Influencer Culture
- Culinary Innovation
- Changing Consumer Trends
- Health Concerns and Considerations
- The Economic Impact
- Cultural and Social Factors
- The Role of Technology
- Government Initiatives and Policies
- Challenges and Criticisms
- Impact on Food Systems
- Veganism as a Social Movement
- Future Prospects

Health Benefits of Plant-Based Diets:

Exploring The Research Behind The Rise Of Veganism And Its Positive Impact On Overall Health And Well-Being.

1. **Reduced Risk of Chronic Diseases:** Examining studies linking plant-based diets to a lower risk of chronic conditions such as heart disease, type 2 diabetes, certain cancers, and hypertension.

2. **Weight Management and Obesity Prevention:** Exploring how plant-based diets, rich in fiber and low in saturated fats, can contribute to weight loss, weight management, and reducing the risk of obesity.

3. **Improved Heart Health:** Discussing research indicating that plant-based diets, especially when they are low in

added sugars and refined grains, can lower cholesterol levels, blood pressure, and the risk of cardiovascular diseases.

4. **Enhanced Gut Health:** Exploring the impact of plant-based diets on the gut microbiome, including increased diversity, improved digestion, and reduced inflammation.

5. **Lowered Risk of Metabolic Syndrome:** Examining evidence suggesting that plant-based diets can help prevent and manage metabolic syndrome, a cluster of conditions including high blood pressure, high blood sugar, excess body fat, and abnormal cholesterol levels.

6. **Reduced Inflammation:** Discuss the anti-inflammatory properties of plant-based diets, which can help alleviate symptoms of inflammatory conditions such as arthritis and promote overall well-being.

7. **Nutrient Density and Adequacy:**
Highlighting how well-planned plant-based diets can provide all essential nutrients, including protein, iron, calcium, omega-3 fatty acids, and vitamins, while being lower in saturated fats and cholesterol.

8. **Improved Digestive Health:**
Exploring how plant-based diets, rich in fiber and prebiotics, can support a healthy digestive system, prevent constipation, and reduce the risk of gastrointestinal disorders.

9. **Antioxidant Protection:** Discuss the abundance of antioxidants found in plant-based foods, which help protect against oxidative stress, cellular damage, and age-related diseases.

10. **Potential Mental Health Benefits:**
Exploring emerging research suggesting a possible link between plant-based diets and improved mental health outcomes, including reduced risk of depression and anxiety.

11. **Longevity and Aging:** Examining studies associating plant-based diets with

longevity and healthy aging, including the role of plant compounds in promoting cellular health and reducing oxidative damage.

12. **Athletic Performance and Recovery:** Discussing the benefits of plant-based diets for athletes, including improved endurance, muscle recovery, and reduced inflammation.

13. **Diabetes Management:** Exploring how plant-based diets, particularly those high in whole grains, legumes, and fiber, can be beneficial for individuals with type 2 diabetes in managing blood sugar levels.

14. **Skin Health:** Highlighting the potential positive effects of plant-based diets on skin health, including a reduction in acne, improved skin elasticity, and a youthful complexion.

15. **Overall Well-being and Quality of Life:** Discussing the holistic benefits of plant-based diets on physical, mental, and emotional well-being, contributing to an improved quality of life.

Environmental Implications:

Discuss The Environmental Reasons For The Popularity Of Plant-Based Diets, Including Reducing Greenhouse Gas Emissions, Deforestation, And Water Consumption.

1. **Greenhouse Gas Emissions:** Exploring how plant-based diets can significantly reduce greenhouse gas emissions compared to animal-based diets, as livestock farming contributes significantly to methane and nitrous oxide emissions, both potent greenhouse gasses.

2. **Land Use and Deforestation:** Discussing the link between animal agriculture and deforestation, as vast amounts of land are cleared for livestock grazing and growing animal feed crops, leading to habitat loss, biodiversity

decline, and carbon dioxide release from forest destruction.

3. **Water Conservation:** Examining the water-intensive nature of animal agriculture, where large quantities of water are required for animal hydration, feed production, and processing, and how transitioning to plant-based diets can help conserve water resources.

4. **Soil Degradation and Erosion:** Exploring the impact of intensive animal farming practices on soil health, including nutrient depletion, soil erosion, and contamination from manure runoff, and how plant-based diets can mitigate these issues.

5. **Water Pollution:** Discussing the pollution of water bodies caused by runoff from animal farms, containing excess nutrients, antibiotics, hormones, and pathogens, and how reducing animal agriculture can help protect water quality.

6. **Fossil Fuel Dependency:** Examining the energy-intensive processes involved in animal farming, including feed production, transportation, and processing, and how transitioning to plant-based diets can reduce reliance on fossil fuels.

7. **Biodiversity Conservation:** Highlighting the connection between animal agriculture and biodiversity loss, as the expansion of livestock production often leads to the destruction of natural habitats, threatening vulnerable species and ecosystems.

8. **Antibiotic Resistance:** Discussing the overuse of antibiotics in animal agriculture and its contribution to the development of antibiotic-resistant bacteria, a significant public health concern, and how reduced meat consumption can help address this issue.

9. **Waste and Pollution:** Exploring the environmental impact of animal waste,

which can contaminate soil, water, and air, and discussing how plant-based diets can help reduce the generation of animal waste.

10. **Climate Change Mitigation:** Discussing the potential of plant-based diets as a climate change mitigation strategy, as reducing animal agriculture can help lower emissions, decrease the demand for intensive agricultural practices, and promote sustainable land use.

11. **Resource Efficiency:** Highlighting how plant-based diets require fewer resources such as land, water, and energy compared to animal-based diets, making them more sustainable and efficient in feeding a growing global population.

12. **Conservation of Wild Fisheries:** Discussing the pressure on marine ecosystems from overfishing, including bycatch and habitat destruction, and how shifting to plant-based diets can alleviate

the strain on wild fish populations and marine environments.

13. **Sustainable Food Security:** Exploring how promoting plant-based diets can contribute to global food security by utilizing resources more efficiently, reducing food waste, and redirecting grain production from animal feed to direct human consumption.

14. **Ecological Footprint:** Examining the overall ecological footprint of animal agriculture, encompassing land, water, energy, and other resources, and discussing how adopting plant-based diets can help reduce this footprint and promote sustainability.

15. **Synergies with Renewable Energy:** Highlights the potential synergy between plant-based diets and renewable energy sources, as transitioning away from animal agriculture can free up land and resources for renewable energy infrastructure.

Animal Welfare and Ethical Considerations:

Examining the ethical motivations behind choosing a vegan lifestyle and the growing awareness of animal rights.

1. **Animal Sentience and Moral Considerations:** Discussing the growing recognition of animals as sentient beings capable of experiencing pain, pleasure, and emotions, and the ethical implications of inflicting harm and suffering on them.

2. **Animal Rights Movement:** Exploring the history and development of the animal rights movement, including the work of activists and organizations advocating for the ethical treatment of animals and the abolition of animal exploitation.

3. **Ethical Dilemmas in Animal Agriculture:** Examining the ethical concerns related to factory farming practices, including confinement, overcrowding, mutilations, and the use of hormones and antibiotics, and how these practices have contributed to the rise of veganism.

4. **Speciesism and Equal Consideration:** Discussing the concept of speciesism, which assigns different moral values to different species, and exploring arguments for equal consideration of all sentient beings, irrespective of their species.

5. **Cognitive Abilities of Animals:** Highlighting scientific research that demonstrates the cognitive abilities and complex social lives of animals, challenging the notion of animals as mere commodities and supporting ethical considerations for their well-being.

6. **Animal Testing and Research:**
Examining the ethical dilemmas
surrounding animal testing and research,
including discussions on alternatives and
the growing demand for cruelty-free
practices in various industries.

7. **Environmental Ethics and Animal
Agriculture:** Discussing the
environmental impact of animal
agriculture and how ethical
considerations extend beyond animal
welfare to include the protection of
ecosystems, wildlife, and future
generations.

8. **Farm Animal Welfare Standards:**
Analyzing existing welfare standards for
farm animals, such as labeling programs
and certifications, and exploring debates
on their adequacy in addressing ethical
concerns.

9. **Animal Liberation and Rights:**
Discuss philosophical perspectives on
animal liberation, including arguments

for granting animals rights, extending legal protections, and ending their use as commodities.

10. **Intersectionality and Animal Rights:** Examining the intersectionality of animal rights with other social justice movements, such as feminism, racial justice, and environmental justice, and exploring the interconnectedness of oppressions.

11. **Veganism as an Ethical Choice:** Exploring the ethical motivations behind choosing a vegan lifestyle, including the belief in non-violence, compassion, and the rejection of animal exploitation in various industries.

12. **Alternative Approaches to Animal Agriculture:** Discuss alternatives to conventional animal agriculture, such as plant-based agriculture, cultured meat, and regenerative farming practices, which aim to address ethical concerns while meeting human dietary needs.

13. **Animal Entertainment and Sports:**
Examining ethical considerations related to animal entertainment, including circuses, zoos, marine parks, and animal-based sports, and discussing the growing awareness and activism against such practices.

14. **Education and Awareness:**
Discussing the role of education and raising awareness in fostering a greater understanding of animal welfare issues, promoting empathy, and encouraging the adoption of ethical lifestyles.

15. **Personal Stories and Empathy:**
Sharing personal stories of individuals who have transitioned to a vegan lifestyle based on ethical considerations, emphasizing the power of empathy and compassion in driving change.

Celebrity Endorsements and Influencer Culture:

Analyzing the role of celebrities and social media influencers in promoting plant-based diets and driving their popularity.

1. **Celebrity Influence and Cultural Shift:** Discussing the impact of celebrities and influencers in shaping public perception and driving trends, including their role in promoting plant-based diets and creating a cultural shift towards veganism.

2. **Celebrity Endorsements and Brand Collaborations:** Examining the partnerships between celebrities and vegan brands, highlighting how endorsements and collaborations contribute to the mainstream visibility and acceptance of plant-based diets.

3. **Social Media and Vegan Influencers:** Exploring the Rise of Vegan Influencers on Platforms Like Instagram, YouTube, and TikTok, and how their engaging content, recipes, and lifestyle choices have popularized plant-based diets among their followers.

4. **Accessible Role Models:** Discuss how the endorsement of plant-based diets by relatable celebrities and influencers, including athletes, actors, musicians, and fashion icons, has made veganism more accessible and appealing to a wider audience.

5. **Creating Awareness and Consciousness:** Analyzing the power of celebrity voices in raising awareness about animal welfare, environmental issues, and the health benefits of plant-based diets, leveraging their platforms to promote conscious choices.

6. **Influencer Marketing and Product Endorsements:** Examining the

effectiveness of influencer marketing campaigns and product endorsements in the vegan industry, showcasing how collaborations between influencers and vegan brands drive product sales and market growth.

7. **Challenges and Recipe Influencers:** Highlighting the impact of social media challenges, such as Veganuary or Meatless Monday, and recipe influencers who share innovative and delicious plant-based recipes, inspiring others to try vegan alternatives.

8. **Amplifying Advocacy Efforts:** Discuss how celebrities and influencers can amplify the efforts of animal rights organizations and environmental activists by leveraging their platforms to spread messages of compassion, sustainability, and social responsibility.

9. **Normalizing Plant-Based Lifestyles:** Exploring how celebrity endorsements and influencer culture help

normalize plant-based diets, challenging the perception of veganism as a fringe movement and positioning it as a mainstream and aspirational choice.

10. **Personal Transformations and Authenticity:** Sharing stories of celebrities and influencers who have embraced plant-based diets and their journeys, emphasizing authenticity and personal growth, which resonate with their followers.

11. **Media Coverage and Public Interest:** Examining how celebrity endorsements of plant-based diets generate media coverage and public interest, creating conversations and discussions that further propel the popularity and acceptance of veganism.

12. **Celebrity Chefs and Culinary Influence:** Discussing the role of celebrity chefs in promoting plant-based cuisine, showcasing innovative recipes and techniques, and influencing culinary

trends towards more sustainable and plant-centric options.

13. **Philanthropy and Advocacy:** Highlight celebrities who actively engage in philanthropic endeavors and animal rights advocacy, using their influence and resources to support organizations and initiatives aligned with plant-based lifestyles.

14. **Addressing Criticisms and Controversies:** Analyzing how celebrity endorsements of plant-based diets are met with both support and skepticism, discussing the controversies and challenges they face in advocating for veganism in the public eye.

15. **Long-Term Impact and Sustainability:** Discussing the long-term impact of celebrity endorsements and influencer culture on the adoption of plant-based diets, considering the potential for sustained behavior change and the importance of holistic sustainability beyond trends.

Culinary Innovation:

Exploring the development of creative and delicious plant-based alternatives to traditional animal-based dishes, contributing to the widespread acceptance of veganism.

1. **Plant-Based Meat Substitutes:** Discussing the development and popularity of plant-based meat alternatives, such as burgers, sausages, and chicken nuggets, which closely mimic the taste, texture, and appearance of animal-based counterparts.

2. **Dairy Alternatives:** Exploring the variety of plant-based milk, cheese, and yogurt alternatives available, highlighting their taste, versatility, and contribution to the growing acceptance of veganism.

3. **Egg Replacements:** Discussing the emergence of plant-based egg

alternatives, including liquid substitutes and powdered options, which offer similar functionalities in baking and cooking.

4. **Seafood Substitutes:** Examining the innovative plant-based alternatives to seafood, such as fish filets, shrimp, and crab cakes, which replicate the flavors and textures of popular seafood dishes.

5. **Artisanal Plant-Based Chefs and Restaurants:** Highlighting the rise of skilled plant-based chefs and gourmet vegan restaurants that offer a wide range of creative and delicious plant-based dishes, showcasing the culinary potential of vegan cuisine.

6. **Plant-Based Fast Food:** Exploring how major fast-food chains have incorporated plant-based options into their menus, providing accessible and convenient plant-based alternatives to traditional fast food.

7. **Global Cuisine Adaptations:** Discussing the adaptation of various cuisines, such as Asian, Mediterranean, Mexican, and Italian, to plant-based diets, showcasing the diversity and cultural richness of vegan culinary options.

8. **Plant-Based Baking:** Exploring the development of vegan baking techniques and ingredients, including egg and dairy replacements, allowing for the creation of delectable cakes, cookies, pastries, and desserts.

9. **Fermented Plant-Based Products:** Highlighting the growth of fermented plant-based products, such as tempeh, miso, kimchi, and kombucha, which offer unique flavors and textures while providing health benefits.

10. **Plant-Based Protein Powders and Supplements:** Discussing the availability of plant-based protein powders and supplements, catering to

fitness enthusiasts and athletes who follow plant-based diets, supporting their nutritional needs.

11. **Plant-Based Condiments and Dressings:** Exploring the range of plant-based condiments, sauces, and dressings available, providing flavors and textures that enhance the enjoyment of plant-based dishes.

12. **Plant-Based Ice Cream and Desserts:** Discussing the development of creamy and indulgent plant-based ice cream options, as well as other vegan desserts like mousse, puddings, and cakes, offering satisfying alternatives to traditional dairy-based treats.

13. **Whole Food Plant-Based Cooking:** Highlighting the emphasis on whole foods and minimally processed ingredients in plant-based cooking, promoting health-conscious and nutritionally balanced meals.

14. **Culinary Innovation in Fine Dining:**
Examining how plant-based cuisine has made its way into high-end restaurants, with chefs pushing the boundaries of creativity and sophistication to craft exquisite plant-based dining experiences.

15. **Home Cooking and Recipe Sharing:**
Discussing the role of home cooks, food bloggers, and online recipe platforms in sharing innovative plant-based recipes, inspiring individuals to experiment with plant-based ingredients and broaden their culinary horizons.

Changing Consumer Trends:

Investigating the shift in consumer preferences towards plant-based products and the impact of this trend on the food industry.

1. **Increasing Demand for Plant-Based Foods:** Examining the rising consumer interest in plant-based products and the growing demand for vegetarian and vegan options in grocery stores, restaurants, and food service establishments.

2. **Health and Wellness Consciousness:** Discussing the role of health-conscious consumers in driving the demand for plant-based products, as individuals seek healthier alternatives and adopt plant-based diets for their perceived health benefits.

3. **Ethical and Environmental Considerations:** Exploring how consumers' increasing awareness of animal welfare and environmental sustainability issues has influenced their food choices, leading to a shift towards plant-based diets and products.

4. **Mainstream Acceptance and Accessibility:** Highlighting the mainstream acceptance of plant-based options and the increased accessibility of plant-based products in supermarkets, online retailers, and food delivery services, catering to a wider consumer base.

5. **Influence of Millennial and Gen Z Consumers:** Analyzing the preferences of younger generations, who are more likely to embrace plant-based diets and actively seek out plant-based alternatives, shaping consumer trends and driving market demand.

6. **Health and Nutrition Education:** Discussing the impact of nutrition education and awareness campaigns that emphasize the benefits of plant-based diets, empowering consumers to make informed choices and driving the adoption of plant-based products.

7. **Flexitarian and Reducetarian Lifestyles:** Exploring the rise of flexitarian and reducetarian lifestyles, where individuals consciously reduce their meat consumption without fully adopting a vegetarian or vegan diet, contributing to the demand for plant-based alternatives.

8. **Social Media and Influencer Culture:** Examining the role of social media platforms, food bloggers, influencers, and online communities in promoting plant-based diets and creating a sense of community around plant-based lifestyles, influencing consumer preferences.

9. **Plant-Based Product Innovation:**
Highlighting the efforts of the food industry in developing innovative plant-based products that closely mimic the taste, texture, and sensory experience of animal-based products, meeting consumer expectations and preferences.

10. **Retailer and Food Service Responses:** Discussing how retailers, restaurants, and food service providers are responding to the growing demand for plant-based products by expanding their plant-based offerings, introducing dedicated sections or menus, and collaborating with plant-based brands.

11. **Market Competition and Investment:** Examining the competitive landscape in the plant-based market, with established food companies and startups investing in research, development, and marketing of plant-based products to capitalize on the growing consumer trend.

12. **Plant-Based Labeling and Certification:** Discussing the importance of clear labeling and certification standards for plant-based

products, providing transparency to consumers and building trust in the authenticity and quality of plant-based offerings.

13. **Economic Implications:** Analyzing the economic impact of the shift towards plant-based products, including job creation in the plant-based industry, changes in agricultural practices, and shifts in market dynamics for traditional animal-based products.

14. **Influence on Supply Chains:** Examining how the increasing demand for plant-based products has influenced supply chains, including shifts in ingredient sourcing, production processes, and distribution networks, as well as collaborations between traditional and plant-based food companies.

15. **Future Growth and Market Projections:** Discussing the projected growth of the plant-based market, considering factors such as changing consumer demographics, regulatory developments, technological advancements, and evolving consumer preferences.

Health Concerns and Considerations:

Addressing potential nutritional challenges of a vegan diet and providing guidance on meeting essential nutrient requirements.

---

1. **Essential Nutrients on a Vegan Diet:** Discussing the key nutrients that may require attention on a vegan diet, including protein, iron, calcium, vitamin B12, omega-3 fatty acids, and vitamin D, and providing information on plant-based sources for each nutrient.

2. **Protein Adequacy:** Addressing concerns about protein intake on a vegan diet and highlighting plant-based protein sources such as legumes, tofu, tempeh, seitan, quinoa, and hemp seeds, while emphasizing the importance of variety and balanced meal planning.

3. **Iron Absorption and Sources:** Explaining the difference between heme iron (from animal sources) and non-heme iron (from plant sources) and providing tips on enhancing iron absorption by consuming vitamin C-rich foods alongside iron-rich plant foods like beans, lentils, spinach, and fortified cereals.

4. **Calcium Requirements and Plant-Based Sources:** Discussing the importance of calcium for bone health and providing information on plant-based calcium sources, including fortified plant milks, tofu, tempeh, leafy greens (such as kale, broccoli, and bok choy), and calcium-set tofu.

5. **Vitamin B12 Supplementation:** Highlighting the need for vitamin B12 supplementation on a vegan diet, as it is primarily found in animal-based products, and explaining the importance of maintaining adequate vitamin B12 levels for nerve function and red blood cell production.

6. **Omega-3 Fatty Acids and Plant-Based Sources:** Exploring

plant-based sources of omega-3 fatty acids, such as flaxseeds, chia seeds, hemp seeds, walnuts, and algae-based supplements, and discussing their role in brain health and reducing inflammation.

7. **Vitamin D and Sunlight Exposure:** Addressing the challenge of obtaining sufficient vitamin D on a vegan diet, as it is primarily synthesized in the body through sunlight exposure, and discussing the importance of spending time outdoors or considering vitamin D supplementation.

8. **Planning Balanced Meals:** Providing guidance on meal planning to ensure a well-rounded and nutritionally adequate vegan diet, including incorporating a variety of fruits, vegetables, whole grains, legumes, nuts, and seeds, and considering nutrient synergy for optimal absorption.

9. **Fortified Foods and Supplements:** Discussing the role of fortified plant-based foods, such as plant milks, cereals, and nutritional yeast, in meeting nutrient requirements, as well as considering the use of supplements for

specific nutrients if necessary and under professional guidance.

10. **RDA Guidelines and Individual Variations:** Emphasizing the importance of individual variations in nutrient needs, including age, sex, activity level, and health conditions, and recommending consulting with a healthcare professional or registered dietitian for personalized advice.

11. **Eating Disorders and Veganism:** Addressing the potential link between veganism and eating disorders, discussing the importance of mindful and balanced eating patterns, and emphasizing the need for professional support when navigating veganism in the context of disordered eating.

12. **Long-Term Health Monitoring:** Highlighting the importance of regular health check-ups and monitoring nutrient levels through blood tests to ensure optimal health and identify any potential deficiencies early on.

13. **Cooking and Food Preparation Techniques:** Providing tips on

maximizing nutrient absorption, such as soaking, sprouting, fermenting, and cooking methods that enhance nutrient availability, while also addressing potential antinutrients in plant-based foods.

14. **Education and Resources:** Recommending reliable sources of information, such as registered dietitians specializing in plant-based nutrition, authoritative websites, and evidence-based books, to educate oneself about meeting nutrient requirements on a vegan diet.

15. **Balanced Vegan Diets for All Life Stages:** Addressing concerns about vegan diets for different life stages, including pregnancy, lactation, infancy, childhood, and older adulthood, and emphasizing the importance of appropriate planning

The Economic Impact:

Examining the economic implications of the growing popularity of plant-based diets, including the rise of vegan food businesses and investment in alternative protein sources.

1. **Growth of the Plant-Based Market:** Discussing the significant growth of the plant-based market and its positive economic impact, including increased sales and revenue for plant-based food businesses.

2. **Job Creation and Economic Opportunities:** Highlighting the job creation potential within the plant-based industry, from farmers and manufacturers to chefs, marketers, and researchers, contributing to local and global economies.

3. **Expansion of Vegan Food Businesses:** Exploring the rise of vegan food businesses, including plant-based restaurants, food trucks, cafes, and catering services, and their contributions to local economies, employment, and entrepreneurship.

4. **Investment in Alternative Protein Sources:** Discussing the influx of investment in alternative protein sources, such as plant-based meats, cultured meats, and protein-rich plant ingredients, driving innovation and economic growth in the food sector.

5. **Technological Advancements and Research Funding:** Examining the economic implications of increased funding for research and development of plant-based products, leading to technological advancements, improved production methods, and increased market competitiveness.

6. **Supply Chain and Agricultural Shifts:** Discussing the impact of the plant-based trend on supply chains and agriculture, including changes in ingredient sourcing, increased demand for plant-based ingredients, and opportunities for farmers and producers to diversify their offerings.

7. **Retail Industry Transformation:** Exploring how the growth of plant-based diets has influenced the retail industry, with supermarkets and grocery stores expanding their plant-based product offerings, creating new revenue streams, and adapting to changing consumer preferences.

8. **Trade and Export Opportunities:** Examining the potential for trade and export opportunities in the plant-based sector, as demand for plant-based products expands globally, providing economic benefits for countries producing and exporting these products.

9. **Economic Benefits of Sustainable Agriculture:** Discussing how the rise of plant-based diets aligns with sustainable

agricultural practices, including reduced land and water use, potentially leading to economic benefits through increased efficiency and resource conservation.

10. **Economic Resilience and Diversification:** Highlighting the economic resilience and diversification potential offered by the plant-based market, as it provides an alternative revenue stream for traditional meat and dairy producers and reduces reliance on volatile commodity markets.

11. **Market Competition and Consumer Choice:** Examining how the growth of plant-based diets has spurred market competition, with existing food companies diversifying their product portfolios and new players entering the market, resulting in increased consumer choice and economic dynamism.

12. **Influence on Food Prices:** Discussing the potential impact of the growing popularity of plant-based diets on food prices, considering factors such as economies of scale, technological advancements, and shifts in consumer demand and production costs.

13. **Investment in Research and Infrastructure:** Highlighting the importance of investment in research and development, as well as infrastructure for plant-based food production and distribution, to support the continued growth of the plant-based market and maximize its economic potential.

14. **Tourism and Culinary Tourism:** Exploring the economic implications of the plant-based trend on the tourism industry, with destinations and businesses catering to vegan and vegetarian travelers, attracting a new segment of tourists and boosting local economies.

15. **Economic Challenges and Adaptation:** Addressing potential economic challenges associated with the growth of plant-based diets, such as the need for industry regulation, market consolidation, and workforce adaptation, while emphasizing the potential for economic benefits and opportunities in this evolving landscape.

Cultural and Social Factors:

Discussing how cultural shifts and changing societal norms have influenced the adoption of plant-based diets in different regions of the world.

1. **Cultural Perceptions of Food:** Examining how cultural beliefs, traditions, and attitudes towards food influence the adoption of plant-based diets, considering factors such as religious practices, historical culinary traditions, and cultural norms.

2. **Globalization and Cultural Exchange:** Discussing how globalization and increased cultural exchange have exposed individuals to diverse cuisines and dietary practices, leading to the incorporation of plant-based elements from different cultures into local diets.

3. **Veganism as a Social Movement:** Exploring the rise of veganism as a social movement and its impact on cultural perceptions, as individuals and communities adopt plant-based diets to align with their values, ethics, and sense of social responsibility.

4. **Celebrity and Influencer Influence:** Analyzing the role of celebrities, influencers, and cultural icons in promoting plant-based diets and influencing cultural norms, as their actions and endorsements shape public perceptions and behaviors.

5. **Community and Peer Influence:** Discussing how communities, both offline and online, can create a supportive environment for individuals adopting plant-based diets, providing social validation, sharing recipes and tips, and fostering a sense of belonging.

6. **Generation and Age-Related Factors:** Examining how generational

shifts and changing attitudes towards health, sustainability, and animal welfare influence the adoption of plant-based diets, with younger generations often being more receptive to plant-based options.

7. **Education and Awareness Campaigns:** Highlighting the role of educational initiatives and awareness campaigns in promoting plant-based diets, as they help individuals understand the environmental, health, and ethical impacts of their food choices.

8. **Cultural Adaptation of Plant-Based Foods:** Discussing how plant-based diets are being adapted and integrated into traditional culinary practices, with local and regional cuisines incorporating plant-based ingredients and techniques to cater to changing dietary preferences.

9. **Food Accessibility and Availability:** Addressing the influence of food accessibility and availability on the

adoption of plant-based diets, as regions with abundant plant-based options and alternatives tend to have higher rates of adoption.

10. **Health and Wellness Trends:** Exploring how the emphasis on health and wellness in contemporary culture has influenced the adoption of plant-based diets, as individuals seek diets that are perceived as healthier and aligned with current wellness trends.

11. **Food Justice and Social Equality:** Discussing the intersectionality of plant-based diets with social justice and equality, as plant-based diets can be seen as more inclusive and ethical, addressing issues related to food sovereignty, animal rights, and social disparities.

12. **Cultural Resistance and Skepticism:** Addressing cultural resistance and skepticism towards plant-based diets, considering factors such as traditional food habits, cultural

pride, and concerns about the nutritional adequacy and taste of plant-based options.

13. **Culinary Innovation and Fusion:** Examining how culinary innovation and fusion cuisine contribute to the acceptance and integration of plant-based diets into cultural culinary landscapes, creating new flavors and dishes that appeal to diverse palates.

14. **Influence of Traditional Medicine and Ayurveda:** Exploring the influence of traditional medicine systems, such as Ayurveda and Traditional Chinese Medicine, which emphasize plant-based diets for health and well-being, on cultural perceptions and acceptance of plant-based diets.

15. **Cultural Shifts and Future Projections:** Discussing the potential for further cultural shifts towards plant-based diets, considering evolving societal norms, changing attitudes towards sustainability, and the influence of younger generations on cultural practices and traditions.

The Role of Technology:

Highlighting advancements in food technology, such as plant-based meat alternatives and lab-grown meat, and their contribution to the rise of veganism.

1. **Plant-Based Meat Alternatives:** Exploring the development of plant-based meat alternatives, such as burgers, sausages, and nuggets, that closely mimic the taste, texture, and appearance of traditional animal-based products, contributing to the rise of veganism by providing familiar and satisfying alternatives.

2. **Technological Innovations in Ingredient Replication:** Discussing how advancements in food science and technology have allowed for the replication of key ingredients, such as heme (from plants) and myoglobin (from

fungi), which contribute to the meat-like flavor and texture of plant-based alternatives.

3. **Cellular Agriculture and Lab-Grown Meat:** Exploring the emergence of lab-grown or cultured meat, produced through cellular agriculture techniques, which involves growing animal cells in a laboratory setting, potentially providing an alternative to traditional animal farming and contributing to the growth of veganism.

4. **Enhanced Nutritional Profiles:** Highlighting how food technology has enabled the improvement of nutritional profiles in plant-based alternatives, such as the addition of essential nutrients, vitamins, and minerals, to address potential deficiencies and enhance the overall nutritional value of vegan products.

5. **Texture and Mouthfeel Replication:** Discussing the role of technology in replicating the texture and mouthfeel of animal-based products, such as using plant-based fibers, proteins, and emulsifiers to create a meat-like chewing experience in vegan alternatives.

6. **Scale-Up Production and Cost Efficiency:** Exploring how advancements in food technology have allowed for the scale-up production of plant-based alternatives, leading to increased availability, affordability, and accessibility of vegan products for a wider consumer base.

7. **Process and Ingredient Optimization:** Discussing how technology enables the optimization of production processes and ingredient formulations, leading to improved taste, texture, and quality of plant-based alternatives over time.

8. **Consumer Acceptance and Market Demand:** Highlighting the influence of technology in driving consumer acceptance of plant-based alternatives, as advancements allow for products that closely resemble animal-based counterparts, meeting consumer expectations and preferences.

9. **Supply Chain and Distribution Efficiency:** Discussing how technological advancements have improved supply chain and distribution efficiency for plant-based products, allowing for better logistics, storage, and transportation to meet the increasing demand for vegan alternatives.

10. **Innovation and Competition:** Exploring how technology-driven innovations in the plant-based food sector have spurred competition among food companies, leading to continuous product improvement, new product launches, and a wider variety of vegan options in the market.

11. **Culinary Creativity and Recipe Development:** Discussing how technology has facilitated culinary creativity and recipe development in the plant-based space, with chefs and food scientists collaborating to create innovative and delicious plant-based dishes.

12. **Environmental Sustainability:** Highlighting how food technology and the development of plant-based alternatives contribute to environmental sustainability by reducing land use, water consumption, and greenhouse gas emissions associated with traditional animal agriculture.

13. **Future Prospects and Innovation:** Discussing the potential for further advancements in food technology, such as 3D printing of plant-based foods, precision fermentation for ingredient production, and novel processing techniques, driving the growth of

veganism and expanding the possibilities for plant-based products.

14. **Consumer Education and Awareness:** Addressing the role of technology in raising consumer awareness about plant-based alternatives through digital platforms, social media, and online communities, providing information, recipes, and resources to support individuals in adopting vegan diets.

15. **Collaboration and Partnerships:** Exploring how technology-driven collaborations between food companies, research institutions, and startups have accelerated the development and adoption of plant-based alternatives, fostering innovation and growth in the vegan food sector.

Government Initiatives and Policies:

Exploring the role of governments in promoting plant-based diets through policies, regulations, and public health campaigns.

1. **Dietary Guidelines and Recommendations:** Discussing how governments develop and update dietary guidelines that promote plant-based diets as part of a healthy and sustainable eating pattern, providing recommendations and educational resources to the public.

2. **Nutrition Education Programs:** Exploring government-funded nutrition education programs that aim to raise awareness about the health benefits of plant-based diets, providing information

on meal planning, cooking skills, and nutritional adequacy.

3. **Food Labeling and Standards:** Highlighting the role of government regulations in ensuring accurate food labeling, including the identification of vegan and plant-based products, allowing consumers to make informed choices and facilitating the growth of the plant-based market.

4. **Subsidies and Incentives:** Discussing government subsidies and incentives for plant-based agriculture, research, and development, encouraging the production of plant-based foods, alternative protein sources, and environmentally friendly farming practices.

5. **Public Procurement Policies:** Exploring government policies that prioritize plant-based options in public institutions, such as schools, hospitals, and government offices, increasing the availability and accessibility of

plant-based meals and promoting healthy eating habits.

6. **Taxation and Pricing Policies:** Discussing the potential use of taxation and pricing policies to encourage the consumption of plant-based foods, such as lower taxes or subsidies for plant-based products, making them more affordable and competitive in the market.

7. **Food Safety and Quality Regulations:** Highlighting government regulations that ensure the safety and quality of plant-based products, setting standards for ingredient sourcing, production processes, labeling, and packaging, building consumer trust and confidence.

8. **Animal Welfare Regulations:** Exploring government regulations aimed at protecting animal welfare, which may indirectly contribute to the promotion of plant-based diets by encouraging the reduction of animal products in the food system.

9. **Climate Change Mitigation Strategies:** Discussing how

governments integrate plant-based diets and sustainable food systems into climate change mitigation strategies, recognizing the environmental benefits of reducing meat consumption and supporting the transition to plant-based diets.

10. **Public Health Campaigns:** Highlighting government-led public health campaigns that raise awareness about the health benefits of plant-based diets, targeting specific population groups and providing resources for individuals interested in adopting plant-based eating patterns.

11. **Research and Funding:** Discussing government funding for research on plant-based nutrition, alternative protein sources, and sustainable food systems, supporting scientific advancements and evidence-based recommendations related to plant-based diets.

12. **International Agreements and Commitments:** Exploring how governments participate in international agreements and commitments related to sustainable development, climate change, and public health, which may encourage

the promotion of plant-based diets as part of a global effort.

13. **Collaboration with Stakeholders:** Highlighting government collaboration with stakeholders, including food industry representatives, healthcare professionals, environmental organizations, and advocacy groups, to develop policies and initiatives that promote plant-based diets.

14. **Dietary Restrictions in Institutions:** Discussing government regulations or guidelines that address dietary restrictions, including plant-based options, in institutions such as prisons, military settings, and long-term care facilities, ensuring diverse and accommodating meal choices.

15. **Monitoring and Evaluation:** Exploring government efforts to monitor and evaluate the impact of policies and initiatives promoting plant-based diets, assessing changes in consumption patterns, public awareness, and health outcomes, and using the data to inform future interventions.

Challenges and Criticisms:

Analyzing the criticisms and challenges faced by the vegan movement, including accessibility, cost, and societal resistance.

1. **Accessibility and Availability:** Discussing the challenge of accessibility to plant-based foods, particularly in lower-income communities and food deserts, where fresh and affordable plant-based options may be limited.

2. **Cost and Affordability:** Addressing the perception that plant-based diets can be more expensive compared to diets that include animal products, as some plant-based alternatives and specialty items may have higher price points.

3. **Nutritional Adequacy:** Exploring concerns about meeting nutritional needs on a vegan diet, including potential

deficiencies in nutrients such as vitamin B12, iron, zinc, and omega-3 fatty acids, and the need for careful planning or supplementation.

4. **Cultural and Social Resistance:** Discussing cultural and social resistance to adopting plant-based diets, as traditional food habits, cultural identity, and societal norms surrounding animal-based foods can pose challenges to acceptance and implementation.

5. **Taste and Culinary Satisfaction:** Addressing criticisms related to the taste and culinary satisfaction of plant-based alternatives, as some individuals may find it challenging to replace the flavors and textures associated with animal-based products.

6. **Social Stigma and Social Exclusion:** Discussing the social stigma and potential social exclusion faced by individuals following a vegan lifestyle, as dietary choices can sometimes be met

with ridicule, misunderstanding, or
exclusion in certain social settings.

7. **Lack of Education and Awareness:**
   Highlighting the need for greater
   education and awareness about the
   nutritional adequacy of plant-based diets,
   addressing misconceptions and providing
   evidence-based information to the public,
   healthcare professionals, and
   policymakers.

8. **Marketing and Misleading Claims:**
   Addressing concerns about misleading
   marketing claims and greenwashing
   within the plant-based industry, as some
   products may be highly processed, high
   in added sugars or unhealthy fats, and
   not necessarily healthier than their
   animal-based counterparts.

9. **Sensitivity to Food Allergies and
   Intolerances:** Discussing the challenge
   for individuals with food allergies or
   intolerances to find suitable plant-based
   alternatives, as some common allergens,

such as nuts, soy, or gluten, are prevalent in many plant-based products.

10. **Dependency on Single Ingredients:** Exploring the criticism that some plant-based diets rely heavily on single ingredients, such as soy or wheat, which raises concerns about monoculture, sustainability, and potential allergic reactions.

11. **Lifestyle and Dietary Preferences:** Discussing the challenge of accommodating different dietary preferences and lifestyles within the vegan movement, as individuals may have varying reasons for adopting a plant-based diet, such as health, environment, or animal welfare, leading to differing dietary choices and practices.

12. **Transition and Support:** Addressing the challenges individuals may face during the transition to a plant-based diet, including lack of support, limited knowledge of meal planning, and

difficulty finding suitable alternatives, particularly in social and dining-out situations.

13. **Skepticism from Health Professionals:** Exploring the skepticism or lack of support for plant-based diets from certain health professionals, which may stem from concerns about nutrient adequacy, conflicting research, or limited education on plant-based nutrition.

14. **Infrastructure and Supply Chain Challenges:** Discussing the challenges related to infrastructure and supply chain development, including the need for increased production, distribution, and availability of plant-based products to meet the growing demand.

15. **Balancing Individual Choices with Systemic Change:** Addressing the criticism that focusing solely on individual dietary choices may not address systemic issues related to animal agriculture, sustainability, and food justice, highlighting the need for broader societal and policy changes.

Impact on Food Systems:

Investigating how the rise of plant-based diets is reshaping food production, supply chains, and the agricultural industry.

---

1. **Shift in Agricultural Practices:** Discussing how the rise of plant-based diets is influencing agricultural practices, with farmers and food producers diversifying their crops and exploring plant-based alternatives to cater to changing consumer demands.

2. **Decreased Demand for Animal-Based Agriculture:** Addressing the impact of plant-based diets on the demand for animal-based agriculture, potentially leading to a reduction in livestock farming, changes in feed production, and a shift in land use from animal feed crops to plant-based food crops.

3. **Sustainable Farming Practices:** Exploring how the adoption of

plant-based diets encourages the implementation of sustainable farming practices, such as organic farming, regenerative agriculture, and reduced use of pesticides and fertilizers, to meet the growing demand for plant-based foods.

4. **Supply Chain Transformation:** Discussing how the rise of plant-based diets is driving a transformation in food supply chains, with the development of new distribution networks, increased availability of plant-based products, and changes in retail and restaurant offerings to accommodate shifting consumer preferences.

5. **Innovation in Plant-Based Food Production:** Highlighting how the demand for plant-based foods is driving innovation in food production, leading to the development of new processing techniques, ingredient sourcing methods, and manufacturing processes to create a wide range of plant-based products.

6. **Investment in Alternative Protein Sources:** Addressing the increased investment in alternative protein sources, such as plant-based proteins, cultured

meat, and insect-based proteins, as the food industry adapts to the changing landscape of consumer preferences and sustainability concerns.

7. **Implications for Global Food Security:** Discussing the potential implications of the rise of plant-based diets on global food security, as the shift in production and consumption patterns may require adjustments in agricultural systems to ensure a sustainable and equitable food supply for all.

8. **Opportunities for Farmers and Rural Communities:** Highlighting the opportunities for farmers and rural communities to diversify their income streams by transitioning to plant-based agriculture, producing crops for plant-based alternatives or engaging in agro ecotourism and eco-friendly practices.

9. **Impact on Food Waste and Loss:** Exploring the potential impact of plant-based diets on food waste and loss, as a shift towards plant-based eating may reduce waste associated with

animal-based food production and consumption.

10. **Sustainable Supply Chain Management:** Discussing the need for sustainable supply chain management practices, including efficient transportation, packaging, and waste reduction strategies, to align with the values of plant-based diets and minimize the environmental footprint of the food industry.

11. **International Trade and Market Opportunities:** Addressing the global market opportunities created by the rise of plant-based diets, as countries with competitive plant-based food industries can expand exports and tap into new markets, contributing to economic growth and job creation.

12. **Challenges for Traditional Livestock Farmers:** Discussing the challenges faced by traditional livestock farmers in transitioning to plant-based agriculture, including the need for retraining, investment in new infrastructure, and potential economic impacts on rural communities.

13. **Implications for Land Use and Biodiversity:** Exploring the potential impact of shifting agricultural practices on land use patterns and biodiversity, as the reduction in animal-based agriculture may allow for the restoration of ecosystems, reforestation efforts, and preservation of natural habitats.

14. **Food System Resilience and Adaptation:** Addressing the need for food systems to adapt to the rise of plant-based diets, fostering resilience through diversification, innovation, and a focus on sustainable practices to ensure long-term viability and stability.

15. **Policy and Government Support:** Discussing the role of policy and government support in facilitating the transition to plant-based diets, including incentives, research funding, and regulatory frameworks that promote sustainable and plant-centric agricultural practices.

Veganism as a Social Movement:

Discussing how veganism has evolved beyond a dietary choice and transformed into a social justice movement advocating for a more sustainable and compassionate world.

1. **Animal Rights and Liberation:** Highlighting how veganism as a social movement places a strong emphasis on animal rights and seeks to challenge the exploitation and suffering of animals in various industries, including factory farming, animal testing, and entertainment.

2. **Ethical Considerations:** Discussing how veganism extends beyond personal dietary choices and encourages individuals to consider the ethical implications of their actions, promoting

compassion, empathy, and respect for all living beings.

3. **Environmental Activism:** Addressing the intersection between veganism and environmental activism, as the movement recognizes the significant impact of animal agriculture on climate change, deforestation, water pollution, and biodiversity loss, advocating for sustainable and plant-based food systems.

4. **Social Justice and Intersectionality:** Exploring how veganism as a social movement acknowledges the connections between animal rights, human rights, and social justice issues, recognizing that marginalized communities often face disproportionate impacts from animal agriculture and advocating for a more inclusive and equitable movement.

5. **Health and Well-being Advocacy:** Discussing the promotion of health and well-being as part of the vegan

movement, highlighting the focus on plant-based nutrition, physical fitness, and holistic approaches to health that prioritize both personal and planetary well-being.

6. **Activism and Advocacy:** Addressing the role of vegan activists and advocates who engage in various forms of activism, including grassroots organizing, protests, education campaigns, and media outreach, to raise awareness, challenge societal norms, and promote veganism as a means of social change.

7. **Influence on Consumer Behavior:** Highlighting how the vegan movement has influenced consumer behavior and purchasing decisions, leading to increased demand for plant-based products, the growth of vegan food businesses, and the mainstreaming of veganism in the food industry.

8. **Community Building and Support Networks:** Discussing the importance of

community building and support networks within the vegan movement, providing individuals with resources, information, and a sense of belonging, as well as fostering collective action and collaboration.

9. **Cultural and Social Transformation:** Exploring how veganism as a social movement challenges cultural norms and societal attitudes towards animals, food choices, and consumption patterns, encouraging a shift towards more compassionate, sustainable, and plant-based lifestyles.

10. **Education and Awareness:** Addressing the role of education and awareness campaigns in the vegan movement, providing information about animal agriculture, environmental impacts, health benefits, and ethical considerations, aiming to inspire individuals to make informed choices and participate in the movement.

11. **Collaboration with Other Movements:** Highlighting the collaborative efforts between the vegan movement and other social justice movements, such as environmental activism, feminism, racial justice, and workers' rights, recognizing the interconnectedness of various social justice issues.

12. **Policy and Institutional Change:** Discussing the advocacy for policy changes and institutional reforms within the vegan movement, aiming to create a supportive environment for plant-based diets, animal rights, and sustainable food systems through legislative initiatives, corporate engagement, and government partnerships.

13. **Media and Popular Culture Influence:** Addressing the influence of media and popular culture in shaping the perception and acceptance of veganism, as prominent figures, documentaries, books, and films have contributed to

raising awareness and normalizing plant-based lifestyles.

14. **Veganism as a Symbol of Resistance:** Exploring how veganism is seen as a form of resistance against dominant systems and practices that perpetuate animal exploitation, environmental degradation, and social injustices, embodying a counter-cultural movement challenging the status quo.

15. **Vision for a Sustainable and Compassionate World:** Discussing the overarching vision of the vegan movement, which strives for a future where the well-being of animals, humans, and the planet are interconnected, promoting a more sustainable, compassionate, and just world for all.

Future Prospects:

Speculating on the future of plant-based diets and the potential for veganism to become a mainstream lifestyle choice worldwide.

1. **Increased Global Adoption:** Speculating that as awareness about the environmental, health, and ethical benefits of plant-based diets continues to spread, more individuals worldwide may choose to adopt vegan or plant-based lifestyles, leading to a significant increase in the global vegan population.

2. **Mainstream Integration:** Predicting that veganism will become more integrated into mainstream culture, with plant-based options readily available in restaurants, grocery stores, and food delivery services. This integration may also include collaborations between traditional food companies and vegan

brands to create innovative plant-based products.

3. **Technological Advancements:** Speculating that advancements in food technology, such as improved plant-based meat alternatives and lab-grown meat, will continue to expand, making vegan options more appealing and accessible to a broader range of consumers.

4. **Government Support and Policies:** Anticipating that governments will implement more policies and regulations to promote plant-based diets and address sustainability concerns, such as subsidies for plant-based food production, increased labeling transparency, and educational campaigns to encourage healthier and more sustainable dietary choices.

5. **Collaboration with the Food Industry:** Predicting increased collaboration between the vegan

movement and the food industry, as companies recognize the growing demand for plant-based products and actively work to develop and market sustainable and innovative vegan alternatives.

6. **Education and Awareness:** Speculating that education and awareness about the benefits of plant-based diets will continue to grow, with more emphasis on integrating plant-based nutrition into school curricula and public health campaigns, leading to a more informed and receptive population.

7. **Global Supply Chain Transformation:** Anticipating that the rise of plant-based diets will drive a transformation in global food supply chains, with a greater focus on sustainable and plant-centric agriculture, reduced reliance on animal-based agriculture, and increased investment in alternative protein sources.

8. **Culinary Creativity:** Predicting that culinary innovation in the plant-based space will flourish, with chefs, food entrepreneurs, and home cooks experimenting and creating delicious plant-based dishes that rival traditional animal-based recipes, further breaking down barriers to adopting a vegan lifestyle.

9. **Social Media Influence:** Speculating that social media will continue to play a significant role in promoting plant-based diets, with influencers, content creators, and celebrities sharing their vegan experiences, recipes, and tips, reaching a wide audience and inspiring others to make dietary changes.

10. **Health and Wellness Emphasis:** Anticipating that the focus on health and wellness will continue to drive the popularity of plant-based diets, as individuals increasingly prioritize their well-being and recognize the potential health benefits associated with reducing

or eliminating animal products from their diets.

11. **Improved Accessibility and Affordability:** Predicting that as demand for plant-based options grows, economies of scale and technological advancements will help make plant-based foods more accessible and affordable, reducing the cost barriers that may have previously hindered widespread adoption.

12. **Global Cultural Shifts:** Speculating that cultural shifts will continue to impact the acceptance and adoption of plant-based diets, with younger generations leading the way in embracing more sustainable and compassionate lifestyles, and traditional cultural norms evolving to accommodate plant-based choices.

13. **Climate Change and Sustainability Focus:** Anticipating that the urgency of climate change and sustainability

concerns will further propel the rise of plant-based diets, as individuals increasingly recognize the environmental impact of animal agriculture and seek more sustainable alternatives.

14. **Collaboration with Health Professionals:** Predicting increased collaboration between the vegan movement and healthcare professionals, as the health benefits of plant-based diets gain more recognition, leading to the integration of plant-based nutrition in healthcare guidelines and patient care.

15. **Social Norms and Acceptance:** Speculating that veganism will become more socially accepted and normalized, with reduced stigmatization and societal resistance, as plant-based diets gain wider recognition and understanding as a viable and beneficial lifestyle choice.